SOMATIC EXERCISES FOR BEGINNERS

By Smith J. Offor

Table of Contents

Introduction 7

How Somatic stretching Functions 12

Potential Medical advantages of Somatic stretching 15

Are there dangers associated with somatic stretching. 18

5 Simple Physical Stretches for beginners 20

Standing Awareness 21

2. Hang Your Head 22

3. The Arch and Flatten 23

4. Iliopsoas Exercise 24

5. Carpal Tunnel Exercises 26

Benefits of Somatic exercise 29

Somatic exercise to try 30

Arch and flatten 31

Arch and Curl 32

Washcloth 33

Seated Twist 33

What is the frequency of somatic
exercises? 34

**7 stretching exercises to help you
become more flexible and reduce
stress. 36**

Neck Release 36

Seated Cat-Cow 37

Child's Pose (or Embryo Pose) 38

Supine Spinal Twist 38

Waterfall..................................... 39

Seated Torso Circles..................... 40

Bridge Pose..................................... 40

**How can I incorporate these
somatic exercises into my daily
routine for maximum emotional
benefits? 41**

1. Start your day with a grounding
practice 42

2. Incorporate somatic exercises into
your workout routine 43

3. Take movement breaks throughout
the day 44

4. Use somatic exercises to manage stress.. 45

5. Integrate somatic exercises into your mindfulness practice 46

6. Wind down with somatic exercises before bed.................................... 47

1. How long should I spend on somatic exercises each day? 48

2. Can somatic exercises help with chronic pain?.................................... 49

Are there any specific somatic exercises you recommend for improving emotional regulation?
.... **50**

Deep Breathing: 50

Progressive Muscle Relaxation:........51

Grounding Techniques: 52

Shaking and Tremoring:.................... 53

Somatic Yoga 54

Mindful Movement: 54

Body Sensing:.................................... 55

Slow and Gentle Practice: 55

Breath Awareness: 56

Body-Mind Integration:.....................56

Embodied Meditation:......................57

FAQs **58**

Is somatic yoga suitable for
beginners? 58

Can somatic yoga help with stress and
anxiety? 59

How often should I practice somatic
yoga?..60

**How Do You Practice Somatic
Release?**...................................**61**

Find a Quiet Space: 61

Connect with Your Breath: 61

Body Scan:.......................................62

Gentle Movement: 62

Tune into Sensations: 63

Release and Let Go: 63

Follow Your Body's Wisdom:...........64

Emotional Expression: 64

Integrate and Reflect: 65

FAQs **66**

Can I practice somatic release on my own? 66

How long should a somatic release practice be? 66

Are there any precautions I should take when practicing somatic release? 67

Introduction

Somatic stretching is a practice aimed at releasing muscle tension through natural, unintentional movements. This is especially beneficial for people who suffer from tension in areas such as the neck, lower back, and wrists associated with desk jobs. Before exploring somatic stretching, it is important to understand the concepts of somatics and somatic movements. The term "Somatics" comes from the Greek word "soma" meaning "body". Refers to anything related to or affecting the body. Thomas Hanna is widely credited with coining the term in the context of movement in his 1985 book Bodies in Revolt: A Primer on Somatic Thinking.

Somatic movement is about being consciously present and creating a connection with your body during physical activity. Rachel Tzakor, associate professor of theater movement at the University of Illinois at Chicago and a registered movement therapist, explains that this requires a keen sensitivity to the present moment and movement.

Somatic practice focuses on the internal experience and sensations of movement rather than outward appearance. Somatic stretching can be distinguished from traditional stretching methods. Stretching typically involves deliberate movements and postures that stretch muscles, with the goal of improving flexibility and range of motion. For example, a quadriceps stretch involves standing upright, grabbing the top of one foot, bending the knee, and stretching the quadriceps by pulling the leg toward your butt. In contrast, somatic stretching emphasizes the inner experience and sensation of movement. Sarah Warren, a certified clinical physical educator, explains that it's about using your inner awareness to guide your movements, rather than forcing your body into a certain position. Somatic stretching offers a unique approach to releasing tension and improving mobility. By prioritizing internal awareness and natural movements, it provides a distinct perspective on enhancing flexibility and overall well-being.According to the American Council on Exercise, "somatic stretching" is defined as "moving or holding various parts of the body in ways that extend the muscles." This is different from other types of stretching. The objective is to build adaptability and scope of movement. Think about the quad stretch that your cycling instructor might show you after a ride: standing up, you take the top of one foot, bend the same knee, and pull it up toward your glutes to stretch the quadriceps muscle on that side.

The practice of releasing muscle tension through gentle movement and being aware of how your muscles feel in various positions and movements is known as somatic stretching. It is based on unintentional movements that happen naturally, like stretching when you stand up after sitting for a long time or making circles with your feet when you take off shoes that are too tight. Below, we'll discuss how it works.) Along these lines, numerous physical development experts don't really want to utilize the expression "extending" by any means. Physical adaptability work doesn't really allude to the extending or pulling of muscles, says Sadie Nardini, a Yoga Partnership enlisted yoga educator and the pioneer behind Center Strength Vinyasa Yoga, who is situated in St Nick Barbara, California. Our muscles always release the tensing that they have caused. According to Nardini, "muscles need a deep release of the tension that the brain tells them to hold onto all day and night."

How Somatic stretching Functions

Substantial extending depends on pandiculation, which an article distributed in the Diary of Bodywork and Development Treatments characterized as the compulsory, natural extending of delicate tissues, especially during advances between cyclic organic ways of behaving. In layman's terms, it's the oblivious contracting and delivering of the muscles that occurs during regular developments; one illustration of this is the manner in which we delicately stretch after waking. According to Warren, "the pandicular response is the way that our nervous system naturally releases built-up tension in our muscles." This response is hardwired into our nervous system. They're pandiculating when you see babies and animals stretch and arch their backs.The goal of somatic stretching is to imitate this release of muscle tension. Additionally, there is a lot of tension to release. As a result of stress, trauma, athletic training, injuries, and repetitive daily activities, our nervous system learns to keep certain muscles tight and move in certain ways over time," Warren explains. Although this is intended as a protective mechanism—our muscles contract to prevent overstretching and injury—it can eventually result in suboptimal movement patterns and persistent soreness, tightness, and pain. You must pay attention to how your muscles feel during any given movement or moment when you do somatic stretching. The way to substantial extending is figuring out how to feel the impression of strain in our muscles and different tissues that we've been molded to disregard (a mindfulness alluded to as interoception), says Meredith Sands Keator, the overseer of preparing at Physical Stretch, who is situated in Ojai, California. That requires a great deal of quietness — some of the time, she has individuals come to class and just lie on the floor the whole time. Keator asserts, "Somatic stretching is based on letting the brain slow down and calm down enough to learn the feeling of sensation." It's a particularly tactile encounter. "You don't pull on anything or power any large developments — it very well may be all around as basic as allowing your head to hang and seeing how that feels for different muscles in your neck. You will be able to actively contract and release your muscles once you are able to feel how they feel. This will let go of tension and make you more mobile. "It seems like a dissolving of well established strain, as after the best morning awaken stretch in bed," Nardini says. Think about taking a physical extending course to learn really regarding the way this functions.

Potential Medical advantages of Somatic stretching

While substantial development has been progressively examined and characterized in scholastic writing (especially in its capability to assist with constant agony), there's meager exploration that is taken a gander at the particular advantages of rehearsing physical extending. According to Warren, people who practice it regularly notice improvements in posture, flexibility, range of motion, and balance. In addition, there is research that demonstrates that mobility and flexibility are crucial aspects of fitness that reduce injury risk (particularly for athletes) and promote healthy aging.

The U.S. Branch of Wellbeing and Human Administrations in its Actual work Rules for Americans, for instance, suggests adaptability activities or exercises be important for a normal work-out daily schedule. Managing your overall health can also benefit from the mind-body connection. Assuming you're mindful of how your body is feeling, that implies you're ready to take care of business when something doesn't feel right," says Brenda Rea, MD, DrPH, an associate teacher of family medication and preventive medication at Loma Linda College in Loma Linda, California. You may, for example, notice (when you're focusing) that your neck or back feels more tight than expected. Occasionally, a particular kind of somatic movement, like stretching that area for a little bit longer, might be helpful. different times, you could search out the assistance of a clinical expert to sort out what may be happening, she says. " Having a greater awareness of what you are feeling and experiencing can unquestionably benefit your health." Additionally, there may be a benefit to mental health. Warren explains, "We hold psychological tension in our bodies as well as muscle tension." People may experience less stress overall if they learn to let go of it.

Are there dangers associated with somatic stretching.

Somatic stretching shouldn't be dangerous to you or your health as long as you do it the right way, by paying attention to how different parts of your body feel during each movement and position and never pushing yourself beyond what's comfortable. "The possibly risk is in the event that you're not paying attention to yourself," Keator says, of her experience educating and rehearsing substantial extending. Assuming you're requesting a lot of yourself in a manner that becomes baffling to you, you're probable not going to have the option to achieve the advantages of substantial extending (delivering pressure and solid strain), and you could gamble with deteriorating your temperament. However, if you have a medical condition, illness, or injury that could hinder the practice, consult your doctor first. One caveat is that people who have experienced trauma in the past may not find somatic stretching to be safe. According to Dr. Rea, trauma, particularly adverse childhood experiences (ACES), can result in a disconnect between the mind and body. This detachment fills in as a survival strategy. While it's possible to overcome past trauma and regain the ability to listen to your body, Reah recommends working with a trained, trauma-informed mental health counselor. The right professional will help you understand how past events affect both your mental health and physical sensations, and seek help if you feel unwell at the same time.

5 Simple Physical Stretches for beginners

Assuming you're interested about physical extending, the following are five fledgling agreeable substantial activities to attempt. To increase awareness of how your muscles feel and possibly reap the cumulative benefits of releasing tension, Warren suggests performing each for approximately five minutes and repeating it daily.

Standing Awareness
Warren suggests simply standing and paying attention to various body muscles before beginning any other somatic stretches. Stand up straight with your feet established and notice how your feet hold the floor, she says. Make an effort to tense and relax those foot muscles. Take full breaths and notice how your muscular strength extend and contract, carrying attention to how this feels. Last but not least, take a body scan from top to bottom, paying particular attention to any areas of tension and how your various muscles feel.

2. Hang Your Head

According to Keator, stand up straight with your feet firmly planted on the ground. Gradually look down, allowing it to fall as far down as it will easily go. Take note of how your neck muscles are feeling as you do this. Additionally, take note of how the movement of your neck has impacted nearby tissues, joints, and muscles, such as those in your shoulders and upper back. Take a look at an area of your body that feels tense, such as the back of your neck, and really think about how that tension feels. Notice how it feels to sink into the stretch. Make an effort to let some of the tension go.

3. The Arch and Flatten

Warren suggests doing the arch and flatten if you're having back pain because it lets you release and then regain control of the muscles in your lower back and abdominals. It's a sluggish development done lying on the floor. With knees bent, stand with feet flat on the ground and hip distance apart. Take a full breath, seeing how the muscles in your lower back and abs move as you do. Delicately curve your back, bringing your midsection vertical and squeezing your glute muscles and feet into the floor. Stay as long as you like in this place. Then, gradually bring down your back and straighten it against the floor. Slowly repeat the movement while looking for any tension in your

torso's muscles and trying to let it
go. To learn how to move, watch
Warren's video.

4. Iliopsoas Exercise

The iliopsoas is the muscle bunch
that connects your spine to your
legs, and large numbers of us hold
loads of strain in it. This
movement carries attention to
these muscles and the muscles
encompassing them, so you're
better ready to deliver that strain,
Warren says. With your knees bent
and feet flat on the ground, lie on
your back. Behind your head,
place your right hand. Delicately
lift your head as you all the while
lift your right leg, keeping it
twisted, around 6 crawls off the
floor. (This should make it appear
as though you are only using one

side of your body to perform a crunch.) Check for tension in the muscles in your lower back, hips, and legs and note how they feel. Lower your head and leg gently. Repeat, this time with a slight leg straightening as you lift. Rehash these movements gradually and tenderly a few times, then do likewise on the opposite side.

5. Carpal Tunnel Exercises

If you spend a large portion of your day typing on a computer or other device, Warren says this exercise can help relieve tension in your lower back, shoulders, chest, hands, and wrists.

To perform this exercise, lie on your left side, bend your legs in front of him at 90 degrees, and place your head on your left arm (it can be bent or straight). Place your right hand on the floor and place your upper arm over your body with your elbow bent at about 90 degrees. Place your right hand near your left ear and move your right arm up around your head so that your elbow is pointing straight up. Use your hands to slowly guide your head toward the ceiling, pulling the right side of your hips closer together. (This is like a side crunch.) Feel your muscles contract. When you are ready, release your head and lower it as slowly as possible. Repeat this once. Slowly lower your back with your right arm behind your head, with your right elbow pointing toward the ceiling. Place your left arm at your side. Contract your right arm and shoulder together and move the left side of your body up. Release your head and shoulders and lower as slowly as possible. Repeat all these movements on the other side.

Somatic approaches and practices, such as somatic stretching, are generally considered safe. However, they are part of a developing field of study, and further research is necessary to identify optimal practices. If you wish to formally begin somatic stretching, it is advisable to consult your primary care doctor or physical therapist. This is especially important if you have any health issues, medical conditions, or injuries. Additionally, it's essential to understand that somatic stretching involves more than just performing specific stretches regularly. According to Tsachor, it's not solely about the duration of stretching but about retraining your movements throughout the day. It entails integrating body and muscle awareness into your daily routines, tuning in to your body's signals, and engaging in movements that are beneficial and enjoyable. Once you have developed an awareness of the various sensations in your body, you can incorporate this knowledge into your everyday activities.

Benefits of Somatic exercise

Somatic exercise offers numerous benefits to both physical and mental well-being. According to Schauster, these exercises aim to enhance the connection between the mind and body, leading to improved overall health. Regular practice of somatic movements may also result in enhanced posture, range of motion, balance, and flexibility. A 2020 review highlighted somatic exercise as a promising approach for alleviating chronic pain. Further research is necessary to explore its full potential.

Somatic exercise to try

According to Schauster, any physical activity can be transformed into a somatic form by performing stretches and exercises with somatism with great care and precision. Her words imply that yoga, qigong, and meditation are all ancient forms of somatic expression that involve the body and mind. "Both body and movement are somatic in nature, requiring attention to the experience." Her somatic exercises include choosing to move in a way that feels good for the body, monitoring breathing flow and outflow, feeling your muscles tight or relaxed, and connecting with objects like you.

The exercises listed below are considered essential daily movements of the somatic system. Doing them for five to 15 minutes each day is advisable.

Arch and flatten

While lying on your back and knees, aim for a flat and arching lower spine by taking in air as you go up and exhale while you descend. Try it five to 10 times (or less) as slowly and consciously as possible. Positioned on your back, with bent knees and hands behind you, exhale while lifting your head to flatten the arch and curve. Inhale and lower your head while facing the earth. Try it five to 10 times or less, with as little effort and sensitivity as possible.

Arch and Curl

The Curl technique involves curling your body 90 degrees towards the torso, placing your head on the left arm, and then bending bent at the knees. Place your right hand on your head and place your hand near your left ear. Inhale and lower your right foot while keeping your knees in the air. Use your right arm to assist in lifting your head. Imagine jerking under the armpit, but don't you risk it by doing so?

Side curl

Focusing on the abdominal and ribcage muscles. Slowly lower the foot and head while exhaling. Repeat the action three to five times (or as many as possible), flip the leg, and repeat the motion on the other side.

Washcloth

Place your arms on the ground while wearing a washcloth, rolling them in opposite directions as you roll, with your knees each time facing the side that rolls down the floor. Head straight up towards your knees to execute a complete spinal twist. Let go of your hurry and indulge in the effortless stretching. Try it three to 20 times or less, with as little effort and sensitivity as possible.

Seated Twist

With your right hand on the left shoulder and both knees bent, rotate your body to the side facing left three times or more. With your trunk in a straight line, turn left and right three times. Turning your head and trunk in a different direction is required for the complete spinal spin. While keeping your trunk left, raise your face to the ceiling and drop your eyes to ground three times or so. Perform the same action on your opposite body. Execute this task with care and speed.

What is the frequency of somatic exercises?

Given their gentleness, how often can somatic exercises be performed on a daily basis? The Somatic Systems Institute suggests that individuals should allocate five to 15 minutes each day to perform the actions mentioned above. At its core, the practice is rooted in bodily awareness.

Most somatic exercises and practices are less risky than traditional physical activities, as the mover is more sensitive to body sensations, according to Schauster. The body's signals of sufficiency or rest-time are more easily heard. Even so, regulating the body can be emotionally demanding for some individuals and those with a past of emotional trauma. A reliable somatics expert can be advantageous in guiding body-oriented tasks.

7 stretching exercises to help you become more flexible and reduce stress.

These stretches are meant to help you feel how your body moves and feels by paying attention to what you feel in your body. Do each exercise for one to two minutes. Pay attention to how your body feels and move carefully between poses. These exercises are good for getting rid of body tension in the morning, after exercising, or when relaxing in bed.

Neck Release

Sit in a comfortable position and slowly bring your chin down towards your chest while taking deep breaths. Gently move your head to the side so that your ear gets closer to your shoulder, but don't push it. Do the same thing on the other side to relieve tension in your neck. Keep doing this back and forth to help ease the tightness in your neck.

Seated Cat-Cow

Sit on the floor with your back straight, hands on your knees. Then arch your back like a scared cat, and then drop your belly and lift your chin like a cow. Repeat this movement.

Sit on your knees or cross your legs with your hands on your knees. Breathe in, lift up your chest and stretch the front of your body, including your neck if you can. Breathe out, curve your back, and bring your chin to your chest. Do this series of movements to move your spine.

Child's Pose (or Embryo Pose)

This is a comfortable yoga position where you sit on your heels and bend forward, resting your head on the floor.

"Get on your knees and sit on your heels. " Bend over, with your bottom on your heels and put your forehead on the floor. Put your arms next to your legs with your palms up, or stretch them out in front with your palms down. Keep doing the stretch to help your back and feel calm.

Supine Spinal Twist

Lie on your back and keep your legs straight. Stretch your arms out to the sides like a letter T with

your palms facing downwards.
Bend your right knee and move it
slowly to the left, twisting your
back and lower back. Look at your
left fingertips with your head.
Lower your hips to the floor and
do the same thing on the other
side.

Waterfall

Lie down on your back with your
hands touching the floor, palms
facing upwards. Lift one knee up
to your chest and then straighten
both legs, keeping a little bend in
your knees if necessary. Stay in
this position and take a few slow
breaths. To leave, bring one leg up
to your chest and put your feet on
the ground. You can use a block or
do this pose against a wall for
extra help.

Seated Torso Circles

Sit with your legs crossed and put your hands on your knees. Gently twist your upper body in circles to the right while you breathe, then do the same to the left. Focus on moving one part of your body at a time, keeping your bottom on the ground and your legs still.

Bridge Pose

Lying on your back, bend your knees and lift your hips up towards the ceiling. Hold for a few seconds and then lower your hips back down to the ground. Repeat as needed.

Lie down on the floor with your knees up and your feet flat. Keep your toes pointing forward. Put your arms by your side with your palms facing downwards. Push your hands and feet into the floor and lift your hips up to make a bridge shape with your body. Pause and hold your breath for a few seconds, making sure your hips are in line with your knees. Carefully put your hips back on the ground and then do it again.

How can I incorporate these somatic exercises into my daily routine for maximum emotional benefits?

Are you looking to incorporate somatic exercises into your daily routine for maximum emotional benefits? Well, you've come to the right place! In this article, we will explore how you can seamlessly integrate these exercises into your everyday life. Somatic exercises are a powerful tool for improving emotional well-being, and by incorporating them into your daily routine, you can experience their full benefits. So let's dive in and discover how you can make somatic exercises a part of your daily life!

1. Start your day with a grounding practice

What better way to begin your day than with a grounding practice? Before you even get out of bed, take a few moments to connect with your body. Close your eyes, take deep breaths, and bring your awareness to the sensations in your body. Notice how your body feels against the mattress, the weight of the blankets, and the rhythm of your breath. This simple practice can help you start your day with a sense of calm and presence.

2. Incorporate somatic exercises into your workout routine

If you already have a workout routine, why not add some somatic exercises to the mix? Somatic exercises can be a great complement to other forms of exercise, such as yoga or strength training. They can help you tune into your body, improve body awareness, and enhance the mind-body connection. Consider adding exercises like body scans, mindful

movement, or gentle stretches to
your usual workout routine.

3. Take movement breaks throughout the day

Incorporating movement breaks into your day is not only beneficial for your physical health but also for your emotional well-being. Set reminders on your phone or computer to take short breaks every hour or so. During these breaks, engage in simple somatic exercises like stretching, shaking out your limbs, or practicing deep breathing. These brief moments of movement and mindfulness can help you release tension, re-energize, and improve your overall mood.

4. Use somatic exercises to manage stress

Stress is a common part of everyday life, but it doesn't have to consume you. Somatic exercises can be powerful tools for managing stress and promoting relaxation. The next time you feel overwhelmed or stressed, take a few minutes to practice a somatic exercise like progressive muscle relaxation or body scanning. These exercises can help you release tension, calm your mind, and bring a sense of peace to your body.

5. Integrate somatic exercises into your mindfulness practice

If you already have a mindfulness practice, consider integrating somatic exercises into it. Mindfulness and somatic awareness go hand in hand, as both practices involve bringing attention to the present moment and cultivating awareness of the body. Next time you engage in mindfulness meditation, try incorporating somatic exercises like body scans or mindful movement. This combination can deepen your practice and enhance your overall well-being.

6. Wind down with somatic exercises before bed

As you prepare for a restful night's sleep, wind down with somatic exercises to help you relax and let go of the day's stressors. Choose gentle exercises that promote relaxation, such as deep breathing, progressive muscle relaxation, or gentle stretching. These exercises can help you release any tension held in your body and prepare your mind and body for a peaceful night's sleep.

Incorporating somatic exercises into your daily routine can have a profound impact on your emotional well-being. Starting your day with a grounding practice, integrating somatic exercises into your workout routine, taking movement breaks throughout the day, using somatic exercises to manage stress, integrating them into your mindfulness practice, and winding down with somatic exercises before bed are all effective ways to make somatic exercises a regular part of your life. By doing so, you can experience the maximum emotional benefits that somatic exercises have to offer.

1. How long should I spend on somatic exercises each day?

The amount of time you spend on somatic exercises each day can vary depending on your schedule and personal preferences. Even just a few minutes of focused attention on your body can make a difference. Start with a time that feels doable for you, and gradually increase it as you become more comfortable with the practice.

2. Can somatic exercises help with chronic pain?

Yes, somatic exercises can be beneficial for managing chronic pain. By bringing awareness to your body and learning to release tension and relax, you can reduce the impact of pain on your daily life. However, it's important to consult with a healthcare professional for a comprehensive treatment plan for chronic pain.

Are there any specific somatic exercises you recommend for improving emotional regulation?

Absolutely! When it comes to improving emotional regulation, somatic exercises can be incredibly beneficial. Somatic exercises involve using the body to regulate and release emotions. They can help you connect with your physical sensations, release tension, and create a sense of calm. Here are a few somatic exercises that you can try:

Deep Breathing: Deep breathing is a simple yet powerful somatic exercise that helps to calm the nervous system. Find a comfortable sitting or lying position, close your eyes, and take slow, deep breaths. Focus on breathing in deeply through your nose, allowing your belly to rise, and then exhaling slowly through your mouth. Repeat this for a few minutes, and you'll notice a sense of relaxation and grounding.

Progressive Muscle Relaxation: This exercise involves tensing and then releasing different muscle groups in your body. Start by tensing your toes and then slowly release the tension. Move up through your legs, abdomen, arms, and finally to your face, tensing and releasing each muscle group as you go. This exercise helps to release physical tension and promotes a sense of relaxation.

Body Scan: The body scan is a mindfulness exercise that involves bringing your attention to different parts of your body. Start at the top of your head and slowly move your attention down to your toes, noticing any sensations or areas of tension. As you become aware of tension, imagine sending your breath to that area, allowing it to relax and release. This exercise helps to cultivate body awareness and promotes a sense of relaxation.

Grounding Techniques: Grounding techniques are somatic exercises that help to bring your awareness into the present moment. One simple grounding technique is to focus on the sensation of your feet on the ground. Feel the connection between your feet and the floor, noticing the support and stability. You can also try grounding by using your senses, such as noticing the texture of an object or listening to the sounds around you.

Shaking and Tremoring: Shaking and tremoring exercises allow the body to release stress and tension. Find a comfortable standing position and start shaking your body, allowing the movement to flow through your arms, legs, and torso. You can also try standing with your knees slightly bent and allow your body to naturally tremor or shake. These exercises help to release stored tension and promote emotional release.

Somatic Yoga

Somatic yoga combines the principles of somatic movement and traditional yoga, creating a holistic approach to movement and self-discovery. It can be a powerful tool for improving emotional regulation and enhancing overall well-being. Let's delve into the world of somatic yoga and explore its benefits and some key practices.

Mindful Movement: Somatic yoga emphasizes mindful movement, where you bring awareness to the sensations in your body as you flow through yoga postures. It's not just about getting into the poses; it's about feeling and experiencing the movements from within. As you engage in somatic yoga, you invite a deeper connection with your body and emotions.

Body Sensing: Somatic yoga encourages body sensing, which involves paying attention to the subtle sensations and messages your body sends. By tuning in to your body's wisdom, you can gain insight into your emotional landscape. This heightened awareness helps you notice areas of tension, release blocked energy, and promote emotional balance.

Slow and Gentle Practice: Somatic yoga focuses on slow and gentle movements, allowing you to explore the range of motion in your body with curiosity and without force. The emphasis is on quality over quantity, encouraging you to move in a way that feels safe and comfortable. This approach cultivates a gentle and compassionate relationship with your body.

Breath Awareness: Just like traditional yoga, somatic yoga emphasizes the importance of breath awareness. Conscious breathing helps regulate the nervous system, calms the mind, and supports emotional regulation. Integrating breath with movement enhances the somatic experience, bringing a sense of flow and harmony to your practice.

Body-Mind Integration: Somatic yoga fosters a deeper connection between the body and mind. It invites you to explore the emotional and energetic dimensions of your yoga practice, allowing emotions to arise and be acknowledged. Through mindful movement and breath, you can cultivate a greater sense of self-awareness and emotional well-being.

Embodied Meditation: Somatic yoga often incorporates embodied meditation practices, where you bring your attention to different parts of your body, noticing sensations and allowing any emotions to surface. This meditative aspect of somatic yoga supports a non-judgmental exploration of your inner landscape, facilitating emotional release and integration.

Incorporating somatic yoga into your self-care routine can be a beautiful way to nurture your emotional well-being. Whether you attend a somatic yoga class or explore it on your own, remember to approach the practice with curiosity, kindness, and a willingness to listen to your body's wisdom. Allow the gentle movements and mindful presence to guide you on a journey of self-discovery and emotional regulation.

FAQs

Is somatic yoga suitable for beginners?

Certainly! Somatic yoga can be practiced by individuals of all levels, including beginners. It is a gentle and intuitive practice that encourages you to listen to your body's needs and move at your own pace. Starting with a beginner-friendly somatic yoga class or finding beginner-level somatic yoga videos online can help you get started on your somatic yoga journey.

Can somatic yoga help with stress and anxiety?

Absolutely! Somatic yoga is known for its calming and grounding effects on the nervous system. By combining gentle movements, breath awareness, and mindfulness, somatic yoga can help reduce stress and anxiety. It promotes relaxation, releases tension, and cultivates a sense of inner peace and well-being.

How often should I practice somatic yoga?

The frequency of your somatic yoga practice depends on your personal preferences and schedule. Starting with a few sessions per week can be beneficial. As you become more comfortable with the practice, you may choose to incorporate it into your daily routine. The key is to listen to your body and find a practice frequency that feels sustainable and supportive for you.

How Do You Practice Somatic Release?

It's a beautiful practice that allows us to let go of tension and stored emotions in the body. Somatic release involves intentionally releasing physical and emotional stress through movement and awareness. Here's a step-by-step guide on how you can practice somatic release:

Find a Quiet Space: Begin by finding a quiet and comfortable space where you can practice without distractions. Create an environment that feels safe and allows you to fully focus on your body and emotions.

Connect with Your Breath: Take a few moments to connect

with your breath. Close your eyes, take a deep breath in through your nose, and exhale slowly through your mouth. Allow your breath to become steady and calming, grounding yourself in the present moment.

Body Scan: Start by doing a body scan. Bring your attention to different parts of your body, starting from the top of your head and slowly moving down to your toes. Notice any areas of tension, discomfort, or sensation. Take your time and be curious about what you discover.

Gentle Movement: Begin to engage in gentle movements that feel good for your body. You can start with slow and mindful stretches, such as reaching your arms overhead and gently twisting your torso from side to side. Pay attention to any sensations or feelings that arise as you move.

Tune into Sensations: As you continue with the movements, pay close attention to the sensations in your body. Notice any areas of tightness, pain, or discomfort. Instead of trying to push through or ignore these sensations, gently explore them with curiosity and openness.

Release and Let Go: When you encounter areas of tension or discomfort, invite yourself to release and let go. You can do this by intentionally relaxing and softening the muscles in that area. Visualize tension melting away or imagine yourself releasing any stored emotions that may be connected to that tension.

Follow Your Body's Wisdom:
Allow your body to guide you in the movements. Let go of any preconceived notions or expectations and trust in your body's innate wisdom. Move in ways that feel natural and instinctive, tuning into the messages your body is sending you.

Emotional Expression:
Somatic release often involves expressing and releasing emotions that may be stored in the body. If emotions surface during your practice, give yourself permission to express them in a safe and non-judgmental way. This could include crying, yelling into a pillow, or simply allowing yourself to feel and release the emotions through movement.

Integrate and Reflect: After your somatic release practice, take a moment to integrate the experience. Sit quietly and reflect on what you noticed during the practice. How do you feel now compared to before? Notice any shifts in your body, mind, or emotions.

Remember, somatic release is a deeply personal and individual practice. It's important to honor your own boundaries and listen to what your body and emotions need in each moment. If you're new to somatic release, you may find it helpful to explore guided somatic release practices through videos or classes until you feel comfortable practicing on your own.

FAQs

Can I practice somatic release on my own?

Absolutely! Somatic release can be practiced on your own. It's a personal journey of self-exploration and emotional healing. However, if you feel more comfortable, you can also seek guidance from a somatic therapist or attend somatic release workshops or classes.

How long should a somatic release practice be?

The duration of your somatic release practice can vary depending on your needs and availability. It can be as short as a few minutes or as long as an hour or more. The key is to create a regular practice that feels sustainable for you. Even a few minutes of somatic release can be beneficial in releasing tension and promoting emotional well-being.

Are there any precautions I should take when practicing somatic release?
It's important to approach somatic release with self-care and awareness. If you have any physical injuries or conditions, it's advisable to consult with a healthcare professional before engaging in somatic release practices. Additionally, remember to listen to your body and honor your own boundaries. If any movements or sensations feel uncomfortable or painful, modify or discontinue them.

www.ingramcontent.com/pod-product-compliance
Lightning Source LLC
Chambersburg PA
CBHW051845250726

48659CB00006B/2039